Facial Gua Sha for Women

A Beginner's Step-by-Step Guide on How to Use the Tool and Overview of its Use Cases for Facial Beauty and Health

mf

copyright © 2022 Felicity Paulman

All rights reserved No part of this book may be reproduced, or stored in a retrieval system, or transmitted in any form or by any means, electronic, mechanical, photocopying, recording, or otherwise, without express written permission of the publisher.

Disclaimer

By reading this disclaimer, you are accepting the terms of the disclaimer in full. If you disagree with this disclaimer, please do not read the guide.

All of the content within this guide is provided for informational and educational purposes only, and should not be accepted as independent medical or other professional advice. The author is not a doctor, physician, nurse, mental health provider, or registered nutritionist/dietician. Therefore, using and reading this guide does not establish any form of a physician-patient relationship.

Always consult with a physician or another qualified health provider with any issues or questions you might have regarding any sort of medical condition. Do not ever disregard any qualified professional medical advice or delay seeking that advice because of anything you have read in this guide. The information in this guide is not intended to be any sort of medical advice and should not be used in lieu of any medical advice by a licensed and qualified medical professional.

The information in this guide has been compiled from a variety of known sources. However, the author cannot attest to or guarantee the accuracy of each source and thus should not be held liable for any errors or omissions.

You acknowledge that the publisher of this guide will not be held liable for any loss or damage of any kind incurred as a result of this guide or the reliance on any information provided within this guide. You acknowledge and agree that you assume all risk and responsibility for any action you undertake in response to the information in this guide.

Using this guide does not guarantee any particular result (e.g., weight loss or a cure). By reading this guide, you acknowledge that there are no guarantees to any specific outcome or results you can expect.

All product names, diet plans, or names used in this guide are for identification purposes only and are the property of their respective owners. The use of these names does not imply endorsement. All other trademarks cited herein are the property of their respective owners.

Where applicable, this guide is not intended to be a substitute for the original work of this diet plan and is, at most, a supplement to the original work for this diet plan and never a direct substitute. This guide is a personal expression of the facts of that diet plan.

Where applicable, persons shown in the cover images are stock photography models and the publisher has obtained the rights to use the images through license agreements with third-party stock image companies.

Table of Contents

Introduction	8
Background and History	11
The Gua Sha Tools	14
Gua Sha Tools Based on the Material	14
Gua Sha Tools Shapes	17
How do practitioners perform the gua sha technique?	18
How often should gua sha be performed?	20
Uses of Gua Sha	22
Here are some of the uses of gua sha:	22
How Gua Sha Treatment Can Help With Other Traditional Chinese Medicines	27
The Risks of the Gua Sha Technique	30
Women and Facial Beauty	32
Benefits of Using Gua Sha on Your Face	34
Step-by-Step Guide on How to Perform Gua Sha on Your Face	37
Step 1: Choose the right tool	37
Step 2: Prepare your face	38
Step 3: Begin scraping	38
Step 4: Wash your face	39
Step 5: Moisturize and relax	39
Is Gua Sha Right for Me?	41
Gua Sha and Graston Technique	43
Conclusion	45
FAQ	48
1. Can you tell me about gua sha?	48
2. What is the procedure for gua sha?	48
3. Can you tell me about the advantages of using gua	

sha? 48
4. Does gua sha have any potential negative effects? 49
5. How frequently should I have gua sha treatments? 49
6. How long does a treatment with gua sha typically last? 49
7. Is gua sha a useful method for treating the face? 50
8. Who shouldn't have gua sha treatment? 50

References **51**

Introduction

The term "qi" refers to the energy that circulates throughout the body, as described by traditional Chinese medicine. It is said to be responsible for both a person's bodily and mental wellness. It is believed that the kidneys are the source of qi and that it travels through the body in a network of channels known as the meridians. It is believed that there are twelve primary meridians, each of which is associated with a distinct organ. According to traditional Chinese medicine, illness results from an imbalance in the flow of qi. Acupuncture, herbal medicine, and gua sha are some of the practices that are utilized in traditional Chinese medicine to bring about a state of balance.

In Gua Sha, a kind of traditional Chinese medicine, the patient's skin is scraped using a tool that is both smooth and curved to stimulate circulation and has a therapeutic effect. It is believed that the technique dates back to the 7th century, and it is being used today for a range of diseases, including the reduction of pain, the prevention of colds and flu, and the treatment of digestive issues.

When doing Gua Sha, a tool made of jade or another type of stone that is polished and curved is often used. After applying oil to the surface of the skin, the practitioner will scrape the instrument in a manner that is both hard and soft over the surface of the skin. The scrape should not be uncomfortable; nevertheless, some patients may feel bruising following the treatment due to the nature of the procedure.

Gua Sha may have a variety of beneficial effects, some of which include the alleviation of pain, enhancement of circulation, reduction of inflammation, and improvement of immunological function. In addition, Gua Sha may be used to treat respiratory illnesses like colds and flu, as well as digestive issues like constipation and diarrhea.

Gua Sha is a technique that is effective in reducing the appearance of wrinkles and promoting a more youthful appearance in women. Menstrual cramps, menopausal symptoms, and premenstrual syndrome (PMS) are some of the conditions that Gua Sha can help treat.

Gua Sha treatments can be administered on a more or less regular basis, depending on the ailment that is being treated. One or two sessions per week may be all that is necessary for overall well-being. When dealing with more acute illnesses, three or more treatments per week may be required.

When carried out by an experienced practitioner, Gua Sha is usually regarded as a risk-free kind of treatment.

Nevertheless, there is a possibility of bruising as well as other forms of skin irritation. Please contact a qualified medical expert before arranging a Gua Sha treatment if you have any questions or concerns about whether or not this therapy is appropriate for you.

In this beginner's guide, we'll take a deeper look at the following subtopics:

- Background and history of gua sha
- The Gua Sha Tools Materials and Shapes
- How do practitioners perform the gua sha technique?
- The uses of the gua sha technique
- The gua sha technique in conjunction with the other traditional Chinese medicines
- The risks of the gua sha technique
- Women and facial beauty
- Benefits of using gua sha on your face
- Step-by-step guide on how to perform gua sha on your face
- When to know if gua sha is right for you?
- The gua sha and Graston technique's similarities and differences

So read on to learn more about the gua sha technique.

Background and History

Gua Sha is an alternative kind of medicine that most likely dates back to the Paleolithic period. The practice of Gua Sha dates back to this period. At that time, many thought that relieving symptoms or even causing someone to lose consciousness by scraping or stabbing certain places of the body with one's hands, other hard objects or stones could be achieved by scraping or stabbing specific areas of the body with stones.

It is possible that the records of emergency therapy from "Prescriptions for 52 Diseases" will give the earliest glimpse of this therapeutic method that has been unearthed up to this point. During the excavation of the Ma Wang Dui Han tomb in Changsha, Hunan, in 1973, a collection of medicinal manuscripts known as Prescriptions for 52 Diseases was uncovered. These texts are now known as the Ma Wang Dui Han Prescriptions. The location of the tomb was Hunan. It is thought that this book was composed sometime during the Shang-Zhou dynasty, which would place its creation between the years 1065 and 771 BCE. This document has the distinction of being the very first record of Chinese materia medica that is now known to exist.

Gua sha is still used often in China today, and it is also gaining favor in several other nations across the world. Although the history of gua sha varies from country to country, its origins may be traced back to traditional Chinese medicine in every country.

Indonesia: In Indonesia, it is known as kerikan (lit. "scraping method") or kerokan, and it is utilized as a sort of folk medicine by members of individual homes. In the United States, the term "scraping technique" is more common. Chinese concepts of wellness and illness form the foundation of Indonesia's time-honored medical practice. It wasn't until the fifth century that traditional Chinese medicine made its way to Southeast Asia, a development that subsequently affected the medical system in Indonesia.

The people of Indonesia have the belief that kerokan, also known as rubbing, may expel excess cold wind, which is believed to be the root cause of sickness. The influenza virus or the common cold is referred to as Masuk angin, which translates to "the entry of wind" in the Indonesian language.

India: The practice of Gua Sha was brought to India during the beginning of the 15th century, along with the naval campaigns of Admiral Zheng He. There is a long history of Ayurvedic medicine being practiced in India, including the use of medicinal plants. It is thought that Gua Sha can help bring down fevers, purify the body, and make people feel more relaxed. It is believed that the practice of Gua Sha can improve circulation and assist the body in its natural ability to repair itself.

Vietnam: The Vietnamese translation of gua sha is co gió, which originates from China. This phrase may be loosely translated as "to scratch the wind." Vietnam is a country that has a long history of appropriating the cultures and traditions of its surrounding countries. The practice of gua sha is not an exception to the rule that the Chinese have been one of the most significant effects on Vietnamese culture for several centuries. China's contributions to the field of medicine had a significant impact on Vietnam's healthcare system during the 5th and 7th centuries CE. To this day, people in Vietnam utilize Cao gió as a remedy for ailments such as the common cold, influenza, and fever.

Other terms: People who speak English typically refer to gua sha as "spooning" or "coining," but people who speak French typically call it "tribo-effleurage."

At this time, gua sha is experiencing a renaissance in popularity as an increasing number of individuals are interested in investigating alternative forms of medical treatment. In addition to this, it is well known in the world of beauty as a method for making the skin appear radiant and younger.

The Gua Sha Tools

The tools used for gua sha can be crafted from a wide range of materials, such as bone, jade, horn, and even plastic. Additionally, the form of the tool shifts according to the region of the body that is being worked on. Let's take a more in-depth look at the many sorts of gua sha instruments, categorizing them according to the materials used and the shapes they take.

Gua Sha Tools Based on the Material

Gua sha tools can be made from a variety of materials, including bone, jade, horn, and even plastic.

Bone: Bone is frequently used as a component in the construction of gua sha tools. The bone used to make gua sha tools is often buffalo or ox bone, and the tools are frequently carved into a variety of ornate patterns. It is thought that bone gua sha tools are more effective than other types of gua sha tools because, when applied on the skin, they generate deeper pressure and create more friction than other forms of gua sha tools.

It is also believed that using gua sha implements made of bone can aid improve circulation and decrease inflammation. In the beginning, the traditional gua sha instruments were crafted using animal bones; however, this technique is not nearly as common now as it once was.

Jade: Jade is another common material used for the construction of gua sha implements. Because jade gua sha tools tend to have a smoother surface than bone gua sha tools, they are more suited for use on sensitive regions such as the face and the neck. It is also believed that jade possesses therapeutic powers that might assist in lowering levels of tension and anxiety.

Additionally, it is thought that jade can assist maintain chi, also known as life energy, in a balanced state within the body. Because of these benefits, jade gua sha implements are frequently utilized during acupuncture sessions.

Horn: The fact that horn gua sha tools offer several advantages makes them deserving of consideration. The reduced weight of horn gua sha tools in comparison to the weight of other types of gua sha tools makes it simpler to use these tools for longer periods. It is also stated that using horn gua sha instruments provides a mild massage that can assist in the relaxation of muscles and the alleviation of tension headaches.

Obsidian: The use of obsidian gua sha tools has been shown to have several advantages, notably in terms of the skin. When placed directly on the skin, the smoothness of the obsidian stone can assist to lessen the amount of friction that occurs, as well as any associated discomfort. In addition, the instrument made of obsidian can assist in the enhancement of circulation and the promotion of lymphatic drainage.

This, in turn, may assist to decrease inflammation and stimulate the body's natural healing processes. Finally, using an obsidian gua sha tool can assist to enhance the overall appearance of the skin by stimulating the creation of collagen and minimizing the appearance of fine lines and wrinkles. This can be accomplished by rubbing the skin in a circular motion.

Amethyst: The quartz kind known as amethyst is exceptionally hardy and long-lasting. It is also thought to possess a great deal of therapeutic value. Amethyst is supposed to assist enhance the overall look of the skin when it is utilized as a tool in the practice of gua sha. It may assist in minimizing the appearance of wrinkles, puffiness, and dark circles under the eyes. It is also believed that using amethyst gua sha instruments can assist enhance circulation and stimulate cell turnover. As a consequence of this, they are frequently utilized to assist in addressing a wide variety of skin issues.

Plastic: Even though they are the least expensive option on this list, plastic gua sha tools are just as efficient as their metal counterparts. Plastic gua sha tools, when handled appropriately, have the potential to be just as effective as their more costly counterparts. Therefore, if you have sensitive skin or if you are pregnant, you should steer clear of using plastic gua sha toys. This is because there is a possibility that toxins will be released into the body as a result of using these toys.

Gua Sha Tools Shapes

There are a few different shapes of gua sha tools available on the market, each of which is designed for a specific purpose.

The standard shape: The standard gua sha tool is rectangular and has rounded edges. This type of tool is versatile and can be used on both larger and smaller areas of the body.

The Chinese coin shape: The Chinese coin gua sha tool is round with a raised edge in the center. This type of tool is typically used on larger areas of the body, such as the back.

The heart shape: The heart-shaped gua sha tool is especially useful for working on areas with curvatures, such as the neck and face. The tool can also be used on other parts of the body, such as the back, where there are fewer curves. This type of tool is said to help improve circulation and reduce the appearance of wrinkles.

The spoon shape: The spoon-shaped gua sha tool is designed for use on larger areas of the body, such as the back. However, this type of tool can also be used on the face. When using a spoon-shaped gua sha on the face, it is important to be gentle and avoid the delicate area around the eyes.

These are just a few of the most popular gua sha tools available on the market. When choosing a gua sha tool, it is important to consider your specific needs and goals. It is also important to choose a tool that is made from a material that is gentle on the skin.

How do practitioners perform the gua sha technique?

The practice of gua sha, which is a kind of traditional Chinese medicine, consists of scraping the surface of the skin with a smooth, flat item. Gua sha is used to break up congestion and stagnation in the body, which enables the body to heal itself. This is the objective of the practice. The treatment of colds, the flu, and other respiratory conditions frequently involve the use of gua sha.

Any object that is smooth and flat can be used to make gua sha; however, the typical tool for the technique is a soup spoon or coin made of ceramic. The therapist will massage the client's skin using this instrument. This causes the formation of petechiae, which are very small dots that might be red, purple, or blue. These marks are an indication that the treatment is having the desired effect.

The massage therapist will begin by applying lotion or oil to the client's skin. After that, they will gently massage the skin using an instrument that has a smooth edge, such as a coin. Only one direction should be used while making the strokes. In addition to that, you need to apply a reasonable amount of pressure. It is important to continue making these strokes until the skin turns red or "sha" develops. Petechiae, also known as sha, is a form of symptom that indicates that the therapy was effective. They appear as a result of the discharge of stagnation in the body.

After the gua sha treatment is complete, the therapist will massage any excess oil into the skin using circular motions. They may also administer heat to the region to alleviate any discomfort caused by the injury.

The gua sha experience should not be uncomfortable in any way. On the other hand, some individuals may experience a stinging sensation while the treatment is being performed. After the therapist is through massaging the skin, you shouldn't feel this feeling any longer. The usage of gua sha is generally considered to be a risk-free and very successful treatment for a wide variety of illnesses; nevertheless, it must not be performed on parts of the body that are already experiencing discomfort or pain.

How often should gua sha be performed?

The goal of gua sha is to improve circulation while also breaking up congestion in the body. It is frequently utilized as a treatment for the common cold, influenza, and sinus infections. Many people feel that gua sha may boost both their energy levels and their general well-being.

For optimal effects, Gua Sha should be practiced twice and thrice each week. When treating acute disorders, it can be done daily. If you are new to Gua Sha, you should begin by performing the technique once or twice a week and gradually build up to the whole session. Always pay attention to what your body is telling you, and put your faith in your instincts.

Gua Sha can be practiced on any part of the body where there is congestion or obstruction, including the face, the neck, the chest, the back, and anyplace else on the body. It is important to steer clear of any regions of damaged skin, open sores, rashes, or inflammation. Before doing Gua Sha on yourself or anyone else, you should seek the advice of a trained practitioner if you have any questions.

A straightforward and efficient method of healing, Gua Sha may be practiced in the comfort of one's own home with only the barest essentials required. Regular practice of Gua Sha can assist to improve circulation, alleviate congestion and cold symptoms, and enhance energy levels. Gua Sha also helps to treat cold symptoms.

Always pay attention to what your body is telling you, and put your faith in what your gut is telling you. If you are new to Gua Sha, begin the practice carefully and gradually build up to the desired frequency. If you have any queries or concerns regarding self-care methods such as gua sha, you should speak with a practitioner who is skilled in the area.

Uses of Gua Sha

It is believed that by promoting the flow of blood and lymph, gua sha can enhance circulation and speed up the healing process. Gua sha is utilized for the treatment of pain the vast majority of the time; however, it may also be utilized for the treatment of other ailments such as the common cold, headaches, and digestive difficulties. Although there is not a lot of data to back up the claims that are made about gua sha, a few studies have suggested that the procedure can assist to alleviate pain and inflammation.

Here are some of the uses of gua sha:

Treating pain and inflammation: According to traditional Chinese medicine, the Gua Sha method can help break up stagnation and promote circulation. Gua sha is frequently utilized as a treatment for a variety of diseases, including pain and inflammation. Inflammatory disorders including arthritis, carpal tunnel syndrome, fibromyalgia, and tendonitis are expected to benefit particularly well from exercise since it is supposed to reduce pain and improve mobility.

Boosting immunity: It is believed that gua sha can improve immune function by accelerating lymphatic drainage. Lymph is a transparent fluid that plays a role in the elimination of waste and poisons from the body. It is believed that the technique can aid in the treatment of several diseases, including the common cold and the flu.

Relieving stress: It is believed that by increasing circulation and encouraging the body's natural production of endorphins, gua sha can help relieve tension and promote relaxation. In the treatment of illnesses such as anxiety, headaches, and sleeplessness, gua sha is frequently utilized as a supplemental therapy. There has only been a little amount of study done in a scientific setting to determine whether or not Gua Sha is effective; nonetheless, many who have tried it claim that it helps them feel calmer and less anxious after a session.

Relieving fatigue: It is believed that gua sha can help reduce fatigue by improving circulation and assisting the body in eliminating toxins from the system. It is believed that engaging in this activity can assist in the treatment of diseases such as chronic fatigue syndrome and fibromyalgia.

Relieving headaches: Gua sha is said to help relieve headaches by stimulating circulation and relieving tension. The practice is thought to help treat migraines and tension headaches.

Improving digestion: It is believed that the practice of gua sha might enhance digestion by enhancing the movement of blood and lymph. It is believed that the technique might assist ease blockages in the digestive system and break up stagnation in the body. People who suffer from indigestion, bloating, and constipation are claimed to benefit from the technique since it helps relieve those symptoms. Even though there is no proof from scientific studies to back up these claims, a lot of individuals feel that using gua sha can be an efficient technique to enhance digestion.

Treating flu: It is believed that gua sha can strengthen the immune system, increase the movement of lymph, and decrease inflammation. There is a school of thought that holds that gua sha can be used to treat influenza by alleviating the symptoms of the illness and assisting the body in fighting off the virus. Gua sha is a harmless and mild therapy that may bring some comfort to patients who are suffering from the flu, even though there is no scientific proof to support the claims being made about its efficacy.

Detoxifying the body: It is believed that the gua sha technique might assist in the detoxification process of the body by increasing the circulation of blood and lymph. Acne, eczema, and psoriasis are just some of the skin diseases that are said to respond well to treatment with gua sha. Those who subscribe to this school of thought hold the belief that scraping can aid in the elimination of toxins from the body and boost circulation.

Relieving menstrual cramps: It is said that gua sha is particularly useful for alleviating the cramping associated with menstruation. Many women report that they suffer from pain and discomfort during their periods because of impaired circulation. It is believed that the strokes of gua sha might enhance blood flow, which in turn reduces inflammation and provides relief from cramps. In addition, it is believed that engaging in the practice can assist in the regulation of hormones and lower levels of stress, both of which are factors that might contribute to menstruation discomfort.

For skincare: It is believed that gua sha can improve circulation and assist the skin in more effectively absorbing skincare products. It is common practice to utilize gua sha in combination with face massage because of the widespread belief that doing so confers several health advantages. A more youthful look is one of the benefits, along with an enhanced skin tone and a reduction in puffiness. As a cosmetic therapy, gua sha is gaining more and more attention these days, and many professionals in the field of skincare feel that it has the potential to completely disrupt the business.

Gua sha is a therapy that is both safe and delicate, and it may be utilized to bring about the alleviation of a wide variety of illnesses. It is believed that gua sha may strengthen the immune system, reduce stress, enhance digestion, treat influenza, cleanse the body, alleviate menstruation cramps, and improve skin care.

While there is minimal scientific evidence to support these claims, many people who have tried gua sha report feeling calmer and having less stress following a session. This is even though there is limited scientific evidence to support these claims. People who are suffering from a range of diseases may find some relief from their symptoms via the use of the safe and gentle treatment known as gua sha.

How Gua Sha Treatment Can Help With Other Traditional Chinese Medicines

Traditional Chinese Medicine (also known as TCM) has been practiced by Chinese people for many years and is still quite popular today. One of the various techniques that are utilized in Traditional Chinese Medicine (TCM) to treat a wide range of conditions is called gua sha. In traditional Chinese medicine, gua sha is often used with other types of traditional Chinese medicine to treat a wide range of conditions. Traditional Chinese medicine can benefit from the application of gua sha in several different ways, including the following:

Acupuncture: Several medical issues can be helped by combining acupuncture with the use of gua sha as a complementary treatment. It is claimed that gua sha can help lessen pain by improving the flow of energy and blood through the body, which can also assist alleviate discomfort. To cure illnesses like migraines, back pain, and neck pain, acupuncture, and gua sha are frequently used in conjunction with one another.

Chinese herbs: In traditional Chinese medicine, gua sha is frequently used with other Chinese herbs to cure a wide range of diseases. It is claimed that gua sha can help increase the absorption of Chinese medicines, which in turn can benefit the treatment of a range of diseases. When treating illnesses such as the common cold, influenza, and allergies, gua sha is frequently combined with other Chinese herbal remedies.

Cupping: To treat a wide range of medical ailments, gua sha is sometimes combined with the technique of cupping. It is claimed that gua sha can help lessen pain by improving the flow of energy and blood through the body, which can also assist alleviate discomfort. In the treatment of illnesses like migraines, back pain, and neck discomfort, gua sha is frequently used in conjunction with the practice of cupping.

Massage: Massage is only one of the many treatment modalities that may be used with gua sha to help cure a range of illnesses. It is claimed that gua sha can help lessen pain by improving the flow of energy and blood through the body, which can also assist alleviate discomfort. When treating illnesses like migraines, back pain, and neck pain, gua sha is frequently used with massage as an effective treatment method.

Gua sha is a therapy that is both safe and delicate, and it may be utilized to bring about the alleviation of a wide variety of illnesses. It is believed that gua sha may strengthen the immune system, reduce stress, enhance digestion, treat influenza, cleanse the body, alleviate menstruation cramps, and improve skin care.

While there is minimal scientific evidence to support these claims, many people who have tried gua sha report feeling calmer and having less stress following a session. This is even though there is limited scientific evidence to support these claims.

The Risks of the Gua Sha Technique

When carried out by a practitioner who possesses the necessary credentials and training, gua sha is usually regarded as a risk-free treatment method. However, just like any other kind of manipulative therapy, acupuncture comes with a set of potential side effects that you have to be aware of before scheduling an appointment. The following is a list of potential dangers that may be related to the use of gua sha:

Skin bruising: Bruising of the skin is the side effect of gua sha that occurs most frequently among patients. Some people can experience more significant bruising depending on the sensitivity of their skin and the pressure that was applied during the treatment. Although bruises are typically harmless and will fade away within a few days, some people can experience more significant bruising.

Petechiae: Gua sha can also cause petechiae, which are tiny red or purple spots on the skin that are caused by broken blood vessels. These spots are usually nothing to worry about and will clear up on their own within a few days.

Skin infection: Infection is another risk that may be associated with gua sha use. There is a possibility of contracting an infection whenever there is a break in the skin or an exposed wound. This danger can be reduced by ensuring that your practitioner utilizes sterile tools and carefully cleans your skin before commencing the process. This should be done before the procedure even begins.

It is essential to keep in mind that damaged skin or open wounds are not appropriate areas for gua sha treatment. Be careful to inform your practitioner if you have any wounds or scrapes on your skin so that they can steer clear of those areas while they are working on you during the treatment.

In general, gua sha is a traditional Chinese medicine practice that has been used for generations to enhance circulation and alleviate pain. This method is both safe and effective in its use. Before scheduling a session of gua sha, you should be informed of the potential hazards that are involved with the practice, just as you would be with any other form of medical therapy. Before deciding to schedule a session of gua sha, you should see your primary care physician or another qualified practitioner if you have any questions or concerns about whether or not the treatment is appropriate for you.

Women and Facial Beauty

It is challenging to be a woman and to refrain from continually comparing oneself to other women. In particular about the attractiveness of the face. We are the harshest judges of ourselves, and it appears that no matter what we try, we will never be able to live up to the expectations that we have for ourselves. It seems like there is an endless list of things to improve about one's appearance, whether it be getting rid of dark circles or finally attaining that dewy sheen. Let's take a look at some of the many different face battles that women have to fight.

Acne is one of the most widespread face problems that women experience throughout their lifetimes. Several different variables can lead to acne, including hormones, heredity, and even stress. Even though there are several different over-the-counter remedies, there are instances when they just aren't enough. In severe circumstances, you might even need to consult a dermatologist about the condition. Wrinkles are a problem that many people have with their faces. A decrease in the amount of collagen and elastin in the skin is what leads to wrinkles. This can be caused by a variety of factors, including aging, sun damage, smoking, etc.

Uneven skin tone is another typical facial concern that a majority of women have to deal with. This could be the result of several factors, including prolonged exposure to the sun, melasma, or post-inflammatory hyperpigmentation. Last but not least, we have bags under our eyes. Several factors can lead to dark circles around the eyes, including being dehydrated, not getting enough sleep, having allergies, and so on.

Throughout the years, a variety of potential remedies to assist women with their face issues have been presented. Some of these answers are grounded in cultural ideas, while others are grounded in research conducted in scientific fields. Even while no cure is certain to work for every woman, some therapies are successful for the vast majority of women.

Benefits of Using Gua Sha on Your Face

Women have been utilizing facial treatments for several years to improve their complexion and overall look. Women have utilized a wide variety of methods, dating back to ancient Egypt and continuing right up until the present day in Hollywood, in their pursuit of a more youthful appearance. Today, the Western world is beginning to understand the benefits of gua sha for skin care, and the method is growing in popularity as a means to create a young appearance.

Reduce the appearance of wrinkles: Gua sha has gained popularity as a way to reduce the appearance of wrinkles and fine lines. While more research is needed to confirm the efficacy of gua sha for anti-aging, some anecdotal evidence suggests that the practice can help to stimulate collagen production and improve the overall appearance of the skin.

Improves skin tone and texture: Gua sha technique stimulates circulation and promotes lymph drainage, which can improve skin tone, and texture and promote a healthy glow.

Release muscle tension and toxins: The massage technique helps to release muscle tension and toxins that can build up in the skin, giving you a healthier and more youthful appearance.

Reduce puffiness: When performed on the face, gua sha can help to reduce puffiness and promote circulation. It can also help to drain lymphatic fluid, which can reduce the appearance of under-eye bags.

Reduce puffiness and inflammation: Gua sha is a traditional Chinese medicine practice that involves scraping your face with a smooth object to reduce puffiness and inflammation. Gua sha has been used for centuries in Asia for its healing properties, and it is thought to increase circulation and promote tissue drainage. Many people who practice gua sha find that it reduces puffiness, particularly around the eyes, and leaves their skin looking brighter and more radiant.

Helps improve the absorption of skincare products: Additionally, gua sha can help improve the absorption of skincare products. The massage technique helps to open up the pores and allow the product to penetrate deeper into the skin.

Sculpt the face: Gua sha can also be used to sculpt the face, contouring the jawline and cheekbones. When performed correctly, Gua sha can give the face a lift and help to improve its overall appearance.

Release sinus pressure: Gua sha is often used on the face, and it is said to help reduce sinus pressure and relieve pain. Gua sha is thought to work by stimulating the flow of Qi, or life energy, in the body. This increased circulation is said to promote healing and ease pain and congestion.

Many women are now using gua sha as part of their regular beauty routine. Gua sha can be done at home or a spa. If you're looking for a way to achieve a youthful appearance, gua sha may be worth trying. The skincare benefits of gua sha are now being recognized by the Western world, and the technique is becoming increasingly popular as a way to achieve a youthful appearance.

Step-by-Step Guide on How to Perform Gua Sha on Your Face

Although gua sha can be administered on any part of the body, the facial area is by far the most typical location for the treatment. When applied on the face, gua sha can assist to minimize the appearance of fine lines and wrinkles, enhance skin tone, and lessen the look of any puffiness that may be present. Continue reading to get step-by-step instructions on how to perform gua sha on your face.

Step 1: Choose the right tool

There are variations in the quality of the various gua sha tools. Be careful to get a gua sha tool for your face that is fashioned from a smooth, polished stone or ceramic when you are looking for one to use on your face. You should avoid using any tools made from rough stones since they might irritate the skin on your face, which is more fragile. In addition to that, make sure that the edges of the instrument that you choose to use are rounded and not sharp.

Buying a gua sha tool from a respected retailer that specializes in selling skincare or beauty items is the best way to ensure that you get a tool that is of high quality. If you are unable to locate a gua sha tool in your immediate area, there are several excellent choices accessible to you online. Be careful to do your homework before purchasing to verify that you are receiving a good deal on a product that meets your needs.

Step 2: Prepare your face

Before beginning the gua sha technique, it is important to make sure that your skin has received all of the required preparation it requires. To begin, you should wash your face with a gentle cleanser and some water that is lukewarm so that the pores can shut.

After you have completed washing your face, apply a little layer of oil or lotion to the surface of your skin. This will lubricate the surface of your skin and help prevent it from drying out anymore. Because of this, the gua sha tool will be able to glide over your skin more effortlessly and without causing you any discomfort than it would have been able to do otherwise.

Step 3: Begin scraping

When you have the gua sha tool in your hand, begin scraping yourself from the base of your neck and work your way slowly up towards your chin. It is important to make sure that you just use a light amount of pressure as you run the instrument across your skin; the scraping process should not cause you any discomfort.

Continue this motion throughout your entire face, moving in a sweeping manner from the neck up towards the forehead.

After you have finished massaging your forehead, start again at the base of your neck and keep massaging your face in this manner until you have done at least three passes throughout your whole face.

Step 4: Wash your face

After you have finished scraping your face, it is important to wash the area with cool water and a gentle cleanser. This will remove any debris or oil that has been loosened during the gua sha process. After washing your face, pat dry with a clean towel.

Step 5: Moisturize and relax

Apply your go-to face cream or serum after you've ensured that your face is clean and completely dry. The gua sha method may aid to boost product absorption; thus, it is important to make use of a high-quality skincare product to get the most out of it. After receiving a gua sha treatment, it is recommended that you use a nourishing serum or cream to assist in calming and moisturizing your skin. After applying moisturizer, you should sit still for ten to fifteen minutes to give it time to completely sink into your skin before continuing with the rest of your day as normal.

Gua sha has the potential to be an excellent method for achieving younger-looking, more radiant skin if it is performed using the appropriate implements and techniques. A simple skincare treatment like this one can help to improve circulation, decrease puffiness, and lessen the appearance of fine lines and wrinkles. Give it a shot on your own and experience for yourself the incredible benefits that gua sha may bring about!

Is Gua Sha Right for Me?

When conducted appropriately by a trained practitioner, gua sha is usually regarded as safe for most individuals; however, specific precautions should be taken if you have certain ailments or health concerns. Before you use gua sha, you should be sure to get advice from a qualified medical practitioner if you have any of the following conditions:

Bleeding disorders: Gua sha should not be performed on people with bleeding disorders or low platelet counts, as the process can cause bruising and bleeding.

Open wounds: If you have any open cuts or scrapes on your skin, it is important to avoid gua sha until they have healed. Otherwise, you run the risk of infection.

Fragile skin: If you have sensitive or fragile skin, it is important to be extra careful when performing gua sha. Be sure to use a very light touch and avoid any areas that are inflamed or irritated. If you experience any pain or discomfort, discontinue the treatment immediately.

Circulatory problems: If you have any circulatory problems, it is important to consult with a healthcare professional before trying gua sha. The process can cause dizziness in some people, so it is important to be aware of this before starting the treatment.

Heart conditions: Gua sha should not be performed on people with heart conditions, as the process can cause an increase in heart rate.

Pregnant or breastfeeding: If you are pregnant or breastfeeding, it is important to consult with a healthcare professional before trying gua sha. There is not enough research on the effects of gua sha during pregnancy and breastfeeding, so it is best to err on the side of caution.

Those who are taking blood thinners: If you are taking blood thinners, it is important to consult with a healthcare professional before trying gua sha. The process can cause bruising and bleeding, so it is important to be aware of this before starting the treatment.

Overall, gua sha can be a great way to improve circulation and promote relaxation; however, it is important to consult with a healthcare professional before trying this treatment if you have any underlying health conditions or concerns.

Gua Sha and Graston Technique

You could be familiar with Gua Sha and the Graston Technique, but you could be curious about how the two approaches are comparable to one another. The Graston Technique and the Gua Sha method are both types of treatment that include the use of instruments to massage the patient's skin.

The practice of Gua Sha, which is a kind of traditional Chinese medicine, consists of massaging the skin with a blunt instrument. Scrape or rub is what the Chinese character Gua implies, whereas Sha refers to sand or rigidity. Gua Sha is performed to release any congestion or stagnation that may be present beneath the skin. This may aid in the reduction of pain, enhance circulation, and reduce inflammation.

Instrument-assisted soft tissue mobilization is the basis of the Graston Technique, which is a type of treatment (IASTM). IASTM is a form of therapy that involves massaging the patient's skin with specialized devices. Scar tissue and adhesions under the skin can be broken up with the assistance of the devices. This may assist in the treatment of pain, the improvement of range of motion, and the reduction of inflammation.

Some parallels can be drawn between the Graston Technique and the Gua Sha technique. In each of these treatments, instruments are used to massage the patient's skin. Both of these treatments can help relieve pain, as well as enhance circulation and bring down inflammatory levels.

Nevertheless, there are a few key distinctions to be made between the two types of treatment. Gua Sha is a method of treatment utilized in Chinese traditional medicine that dates back hundreds of years. The Graston Technique is a form of treatment that is considered to be very recent, having been established in the 1990s. Practitioners of Gua Sha have experience and training in traditional Chinese medicine to carry out the treatment. Any healthcare worker who has received training in IASTM is qualified to execute the Graston Technique.

Conclusion

Traditional Chinese medicine has made use of gua sha, a method that dates back millennia and has been around for a long time. When performing gua sha, practitioners make use of a wide array of implements, some of which include metal instruments, horns, bone, or stone. The curved blade is by far the most popular kind.

How is the Gua Sha method carried out by practitioners? First, they determine the parts of the problem that require therapy. After that, a lubricant is applied to the skin, and an instrument called a gua sha is used to exert pressure and rub the skin in a circular motion. This results in the skin becoming flushed and developing little red spots known as petechiae. Gua sha is a treatment that may be used for a variety of purposes, including pain relief, inflammation reduction, and circulation improvement. Other forms of traditional Chinese medicine, such as acupuncture or herbal therapy, can be used with the gua sha procedure to provide optimal therapeutic effects.

The bruising and scraping of the surface of the skin are two of the potential adverse effects of the gua sha procedure. On the other hand, gua sha is a risk-free and very effective treatment for a wide variety of illnesses when it is carried out by an experienced practitioner. Gua sha is used by some ladies as part of their cosmetic regimen to help enhance their complexion and decrease the appearance of wrinkles. Gua sha can also help reduce the pain and tension associated with headaches and neck discomfort.

The Graston method and the gua sha technique are comparable in that they both involve the use of pressure and friction to repair damaged muscles and tissues. However, there are some significant distinctions between these two methods to take into account. Gua sha may be done with virtually any object that is flat on one side, but Graston requires specially developed tools with ridges on them to be used. Because Guasha involves greater pressure than Graston does, some people find it to be more uncomfortable. Gua Sha, on the other hand, is a more affordable alternative to Graston that can be done anywhere.

Traditional Chinese Medicine has made use of gua sha, an age-old method, for several decades already. It is stated that the therapy will assist in the discharge of toxins, will increase blood circulation, and will stimulate lymphatic drainage. It is also useful in the sense that it may alleviate pain, it can reduce inflammation, and can restore the health of the skin.

Gua sha is a treatment that is supposed to offer numerous advantages; however, there are also certain hazards linked with the treatment. These concerns should be taken into consideration before considering whether or not gua sha is appropriate for you. It is vital to keep in mind that the outcomes of gua sha might differ from person to person, therefore women need to keep an open mind about whether or not it will enhance the appearance of their skin.

FAQ

1. Can you tell me about gua sha?

A method of traditional Chinese medicine known as gua sha includes using a smooth, blunt object to scrape the surface of the skin in a circular motion. It is believed that the technique will increase circulation by breaking up stagnation in the body, which will then facilitate healing. Gua sha is usually employed as a treatment for aches, inflammation, and even the common cold.

2. What is the procedure for gua sha?

The jade stone or ceramic spoon that is often used in gua sha therapy is an example of a tool that is both smooth and blunt. After applying oil to the patient's skin to lubricate it, the practitioner will scrape a tool across the patient's skin in a manner that is both hard and gentle. The scraping shouldn't be uncomfortable, although it's possible that some bruising will take place.

3. Can you tell me about the advantages of using gua sha?

It is believed that gua sha may enhance circulation, boost healing, and significantly cut down on pain and inflammation.

Additionally, it is believed that gua sha can strengthen the immune system and assist in the treatment of illnesses like the common cold and influenza.

4. Does gua sha have any potential negative effects?

After receiving a gua sha treatment, you can have some bruising, but this is usually just brief and will go away in a few days at the most. It is essential to refrain from rubbing the skin too roughly since this might result in an injury if not avoided. Gua sha is not dangerous for the vast majority of individuals when it is done properly.

5. How frequently should I have gua sha treatments?

The frequency of gua sha treatments will change from person to person according to what that person requires. Some people may benefit from having treatments performed once a week, while others would simply require treatments on an as-needed basis. When determining the frequency with which gua sha should be administered, it is critical to seek the advice of an experienced practitioner.

6. How long does a treatment with gua sha typically last?

The duration of a gua sha treatment typically ranges from ten to fifteen minutes; however, the amount of time may change based on the requirements of the individual.

7. Is gua sha a useful method for treating the face?

It is believed that regular use of gua sha can assist to enhance complexion as well as lessen the appearance of wrinkles on the face. In addition to this, it is stated that gua sha can assist alleviate tension headaches as well as neck discomfort.

8. Who shouldn't have gua sha treatment?

Because of their medical problems or other circumstances, certain people should not have the gua sha treatment. These individuals include those who are pregnant, those who are taking medications that thin the blood, as well as those who have open wounds or illnesses.

References

Debutify. (n.d.). Gua sha 101: All about how to use the gua sha tool. Sublime Life. Retrieved October 19, 2022, from https://sublimelife.in/blogs/sublime-stories/gua-sha-101-everything-you-need-to-know-about-how-to-use-a-gua-sha.

Ewe, K. (2021, May 5). Does gua sha work? What two weeks of trying the beauty trend did to my face. Vice. https://www.vice.com/en/article/g5ggv7/gua-sha-benefits-beauty-skincare-trend.

Gua sha step-by-step tutorial. (n.d.). La Coéss. Retrieved October 19, 2022, from https://www.lacoess.com/blogs/news/gua-sha-step-by-step-tutorial.

How to use gua sha for tension, puffiness, & lymphatic drainage. (2021, January 22). Healthline. https://www.healthline.com/health/beauty-skin-care/how-to-use-gua-sha.

Imelda, J. D. (n.d.). Got a cold? In coin rubbing Indonesians trust. The Conversation. Retrieved October 19, 2022, from http://theconversation.com/got-a-cold-in-coin-rubbing-indonesians-trust-79270.

Is Gua Sha the newest beauty self-care tool? We think so! (2022, June 7). Lifestyle Asia India.

https://www.lifestyleasia.com/ind/beauty-grooming/skincare/is-gua-sha-the-newest-beauty-self-care-tool-we-think-so/.

Scrapping | chinese acupuncture dubai. (n.d.). Retrieved October 19, 2022, from https://kindcare.ae/tcm/scrapping/.

Tang, K. W. (2020). Gua sha: An ancient therapy for contemporary illnesses. WORLD SCIENTIFIC. https://doi.org/10.1142/11519.

Tcm: Understanding the role of the kidney. (n.d.). Retrieved October 19, 2022, from https://www.euyansang.com/en_US/tcm%3A-understanding-the-role-of-the-kidney/eystcmorgans2.html.

TOA, N. H. I. at. (2018, February 1). Instrument assisted soft tissue mobilization | iastm | nasvhille, tn. Nashville Hip Institute at TOA | Thomas Byrd MD. https://nashvillehip.org/iastm/.

Why gua sha is good for you. (2021, June 14). Cleveland Clinic Health Essentials. https://health.clevelandclinic.org/why-gua-sha-might-be-good-for-you/.

www.ingramcontent.com/pod-product-compliance
Lightning Source LLC
LaVergne TN
LVHW011900060526
838200LV00054B/4437